The First Words Lotería Book for Toddlers

ENGLISH-SPANISH BILINGUAL

Libro de Lotería de primeras palabras para niños pequeños

BILINGÜE INGLÉS-ESPAÑOL

Angélica López

Illustrated by Milena Vargas

Copyright © 2022 by Callisto Publishing LLC
Cover and internal design © 2022 by Callisto Publishing LLC
Illustrations © 2021 Milena Vargas. Author photo courtesy of Ruth Ann García Photography;
Ruth Ann García 2021
Series Designer: Amanda Kirk
Interior and Cover Designer: Amanda Kirk
Art Producer: Samantha Ulban
Editor: Laura Bryn Sisson
Production Editor: Nora Milman
Production Manager: Martin Worthington

Published by Callisto Publishing LLC C/O Sourcebooks LLC
P.O. Box 4410, Naperville, Illinois 60567-4410
(630) 961-3900
callistopublishing.com

Printed in the United States of America.

To my husband, Toño, and my boys,

Babo, Chucho, and Toñito,

who are my inspiration to be a better person.

–A.L.

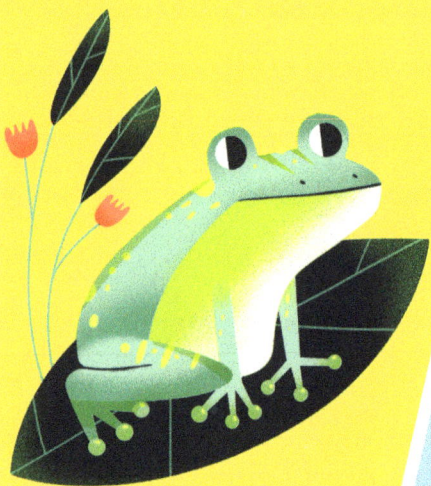

la rana
the frog

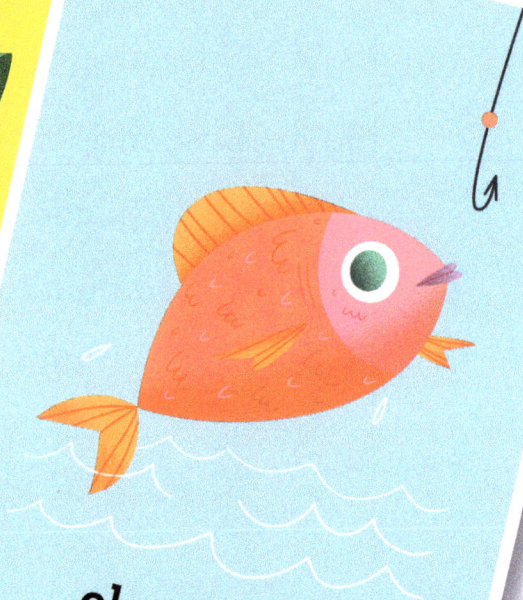

el pescado
the fish

A Note to Parents

La Lotería is Spanish for lottery. Also known as Mexican Bingo, the game *Lotería* is a tradition in Mexico that families have enjoyed for many years. To play *Lotería,* a caller calls out the names of cards, or **cartas,** as they are dealt. When the players have a matching card on their *Lotería* board, or **tabla,** they mark the card on their board. The first player who has 4 marked cards on a vertical, horizontal, or diagonal line shouts *¡Lotería!* and wins the game.

    This book features 44 words and illustrations drawn from traditional *Lotería* cards, which are split into 4 sections: animals, people & music, the natural world, and objects. Each card includes the Spanish name and an English translation, as a fun way for your child to learn their first bilingual words!

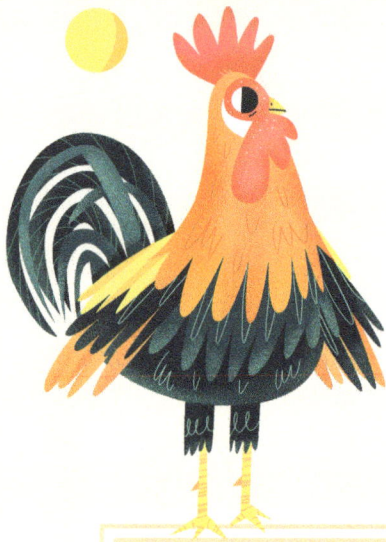

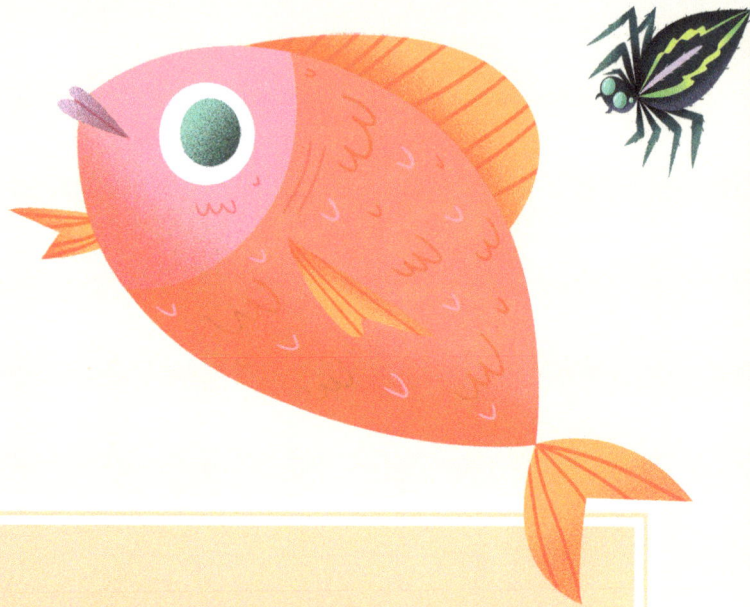

Los animales
Animals

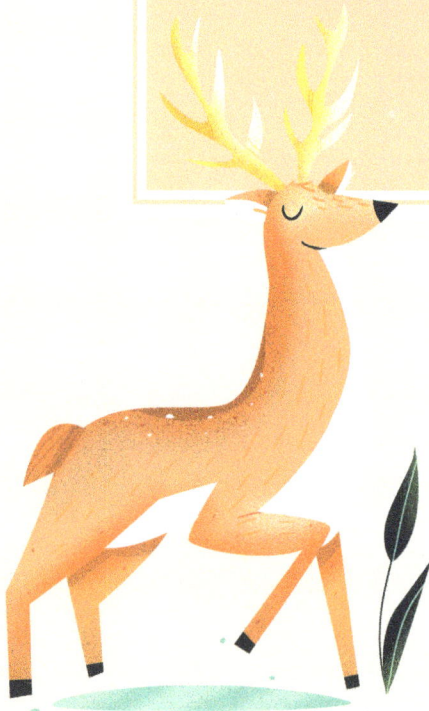

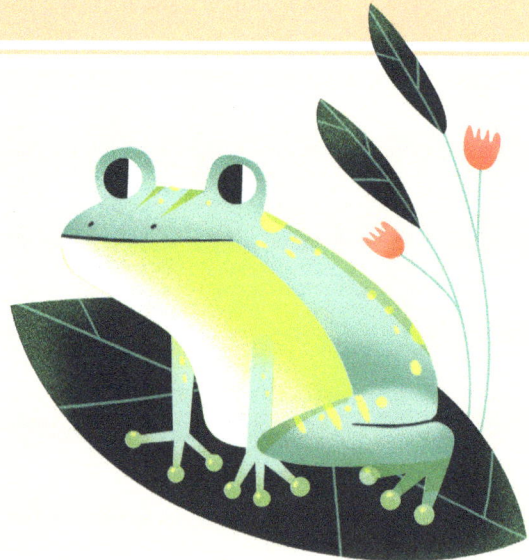

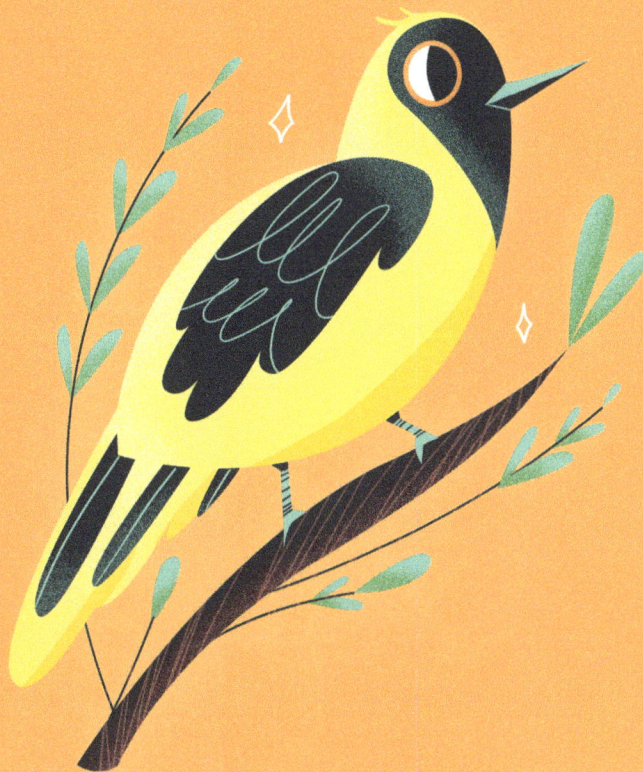

el pájaro

the bird

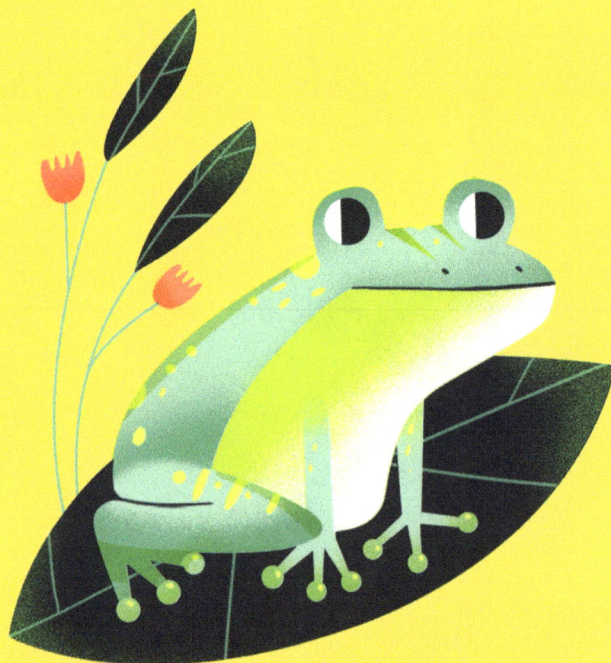

la rana

the frog

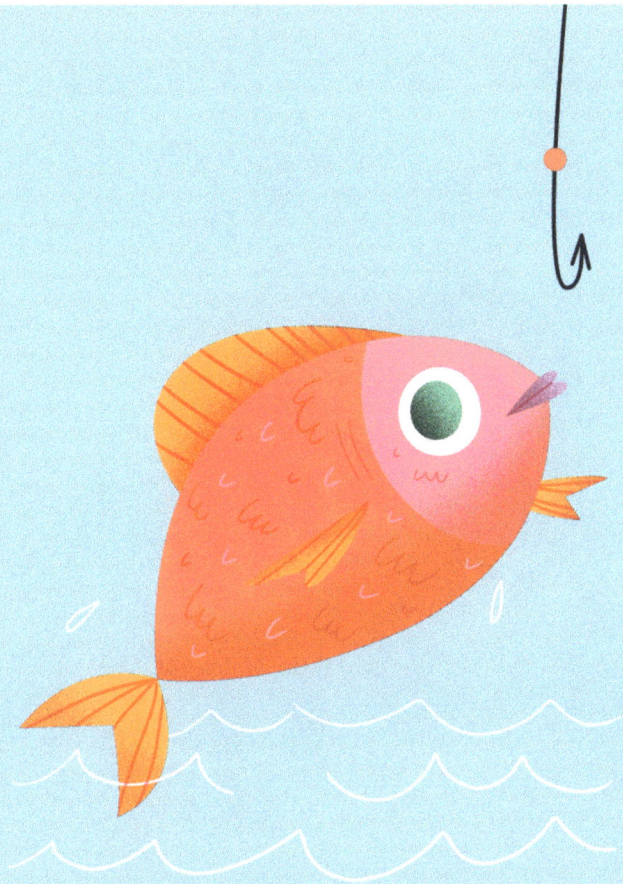

el pescado
the fish

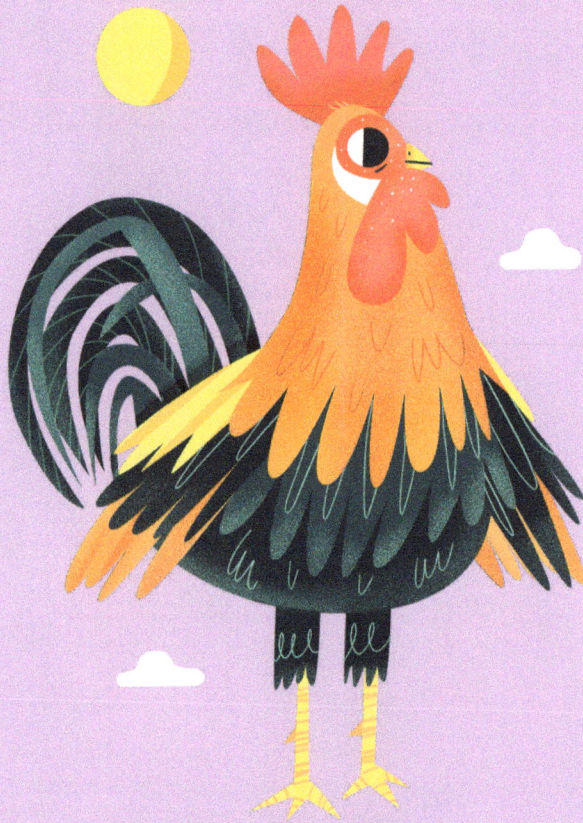

el gallo
the rooster

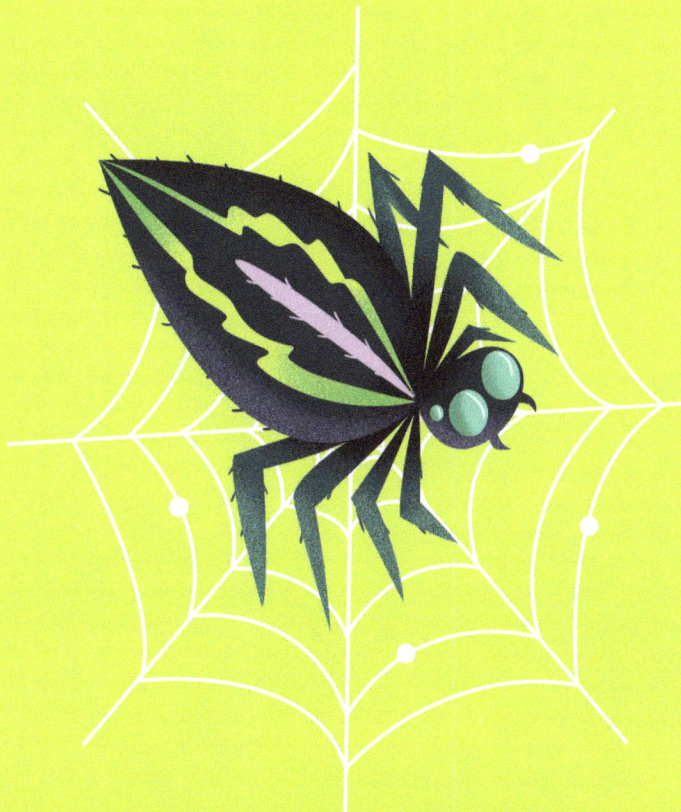

la araña

the spider

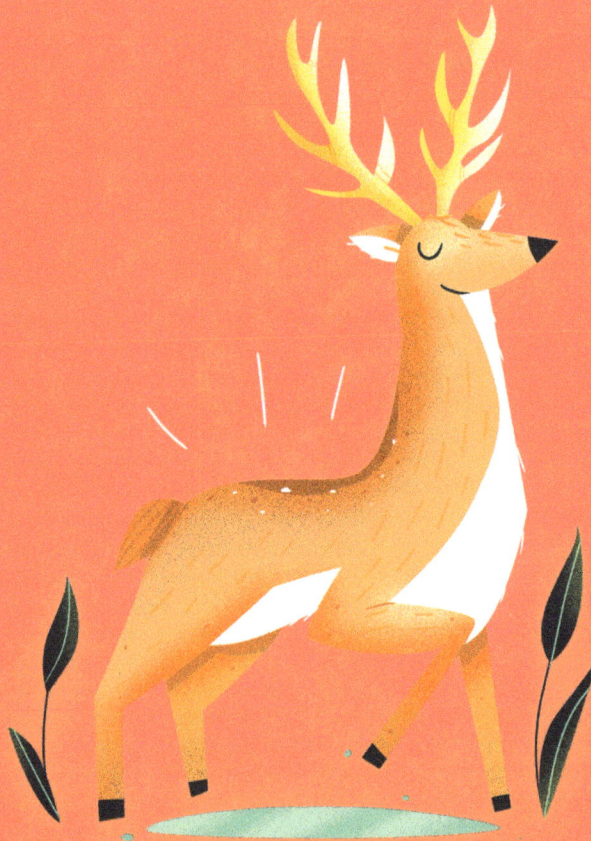

el venado

the deer

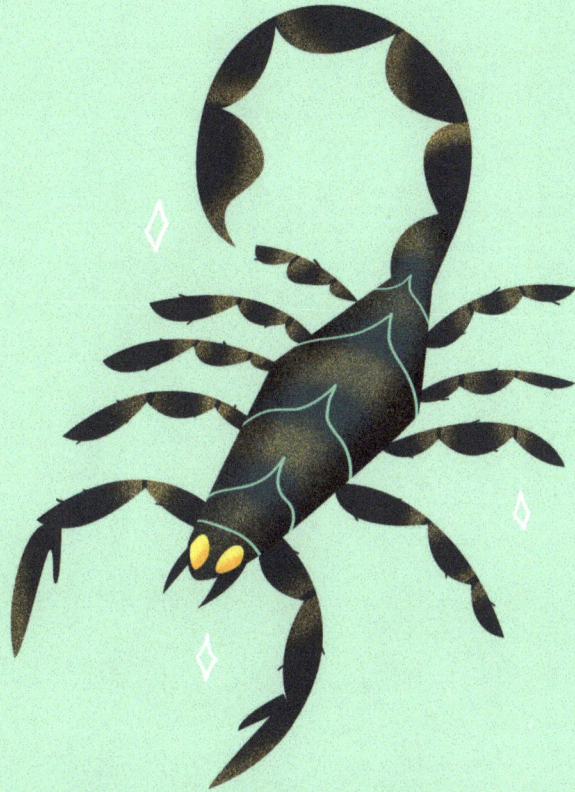

el alacrán

the scorpion

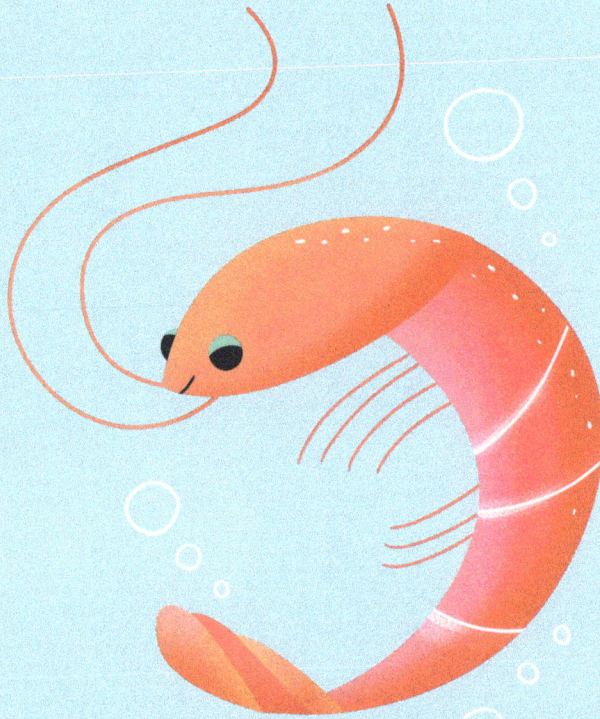

el camarón

the shrimp

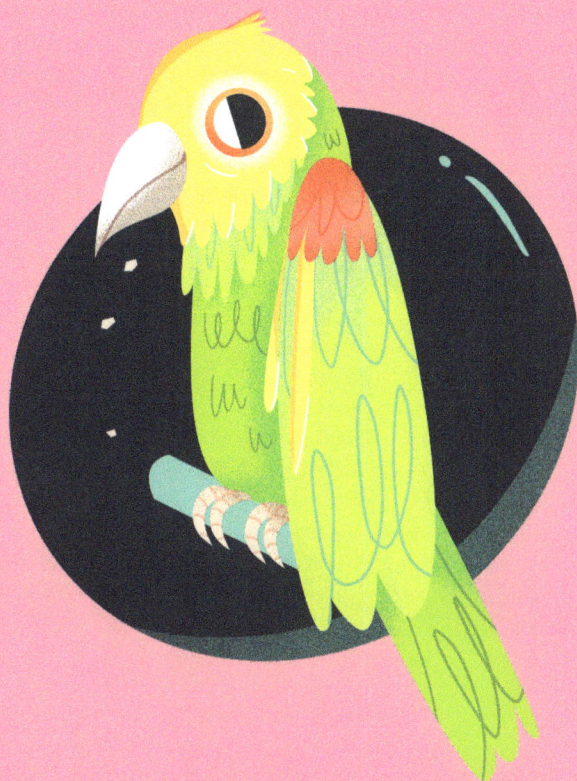

el cotorro

the parrot

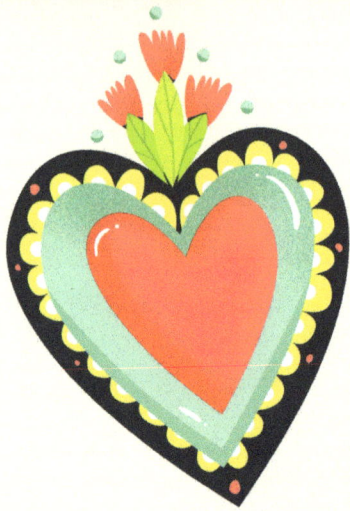

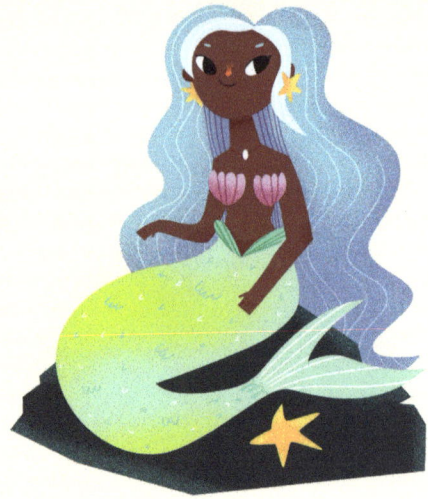

Las personas y la música
People and Music

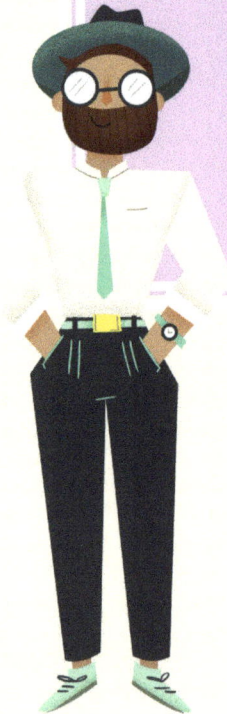

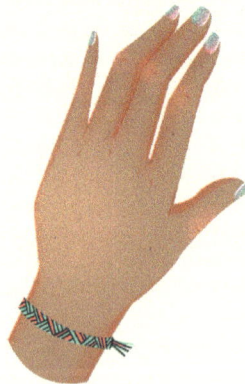

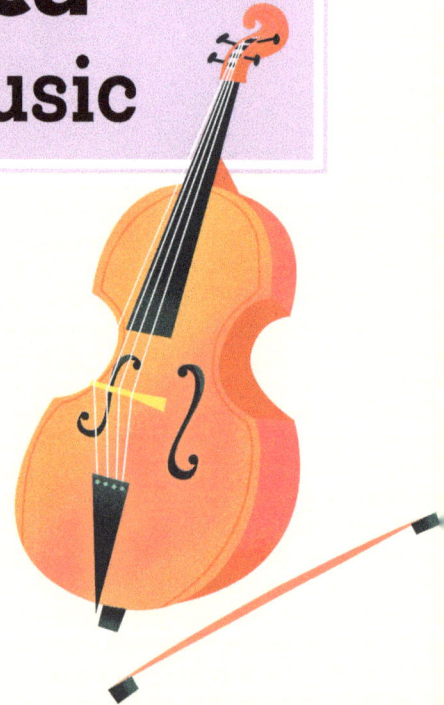

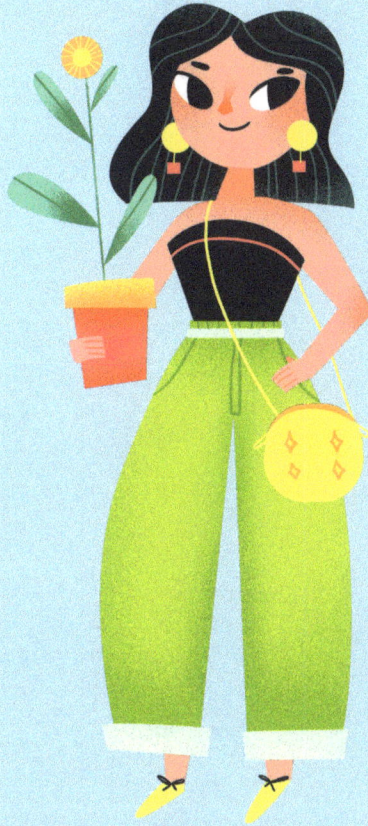

la dama

the lady

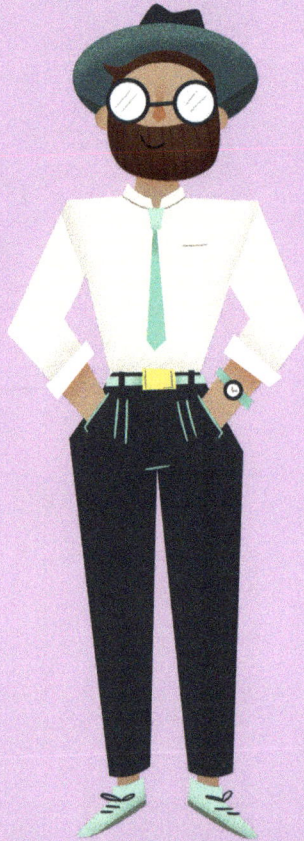

el catrín
the gentleman

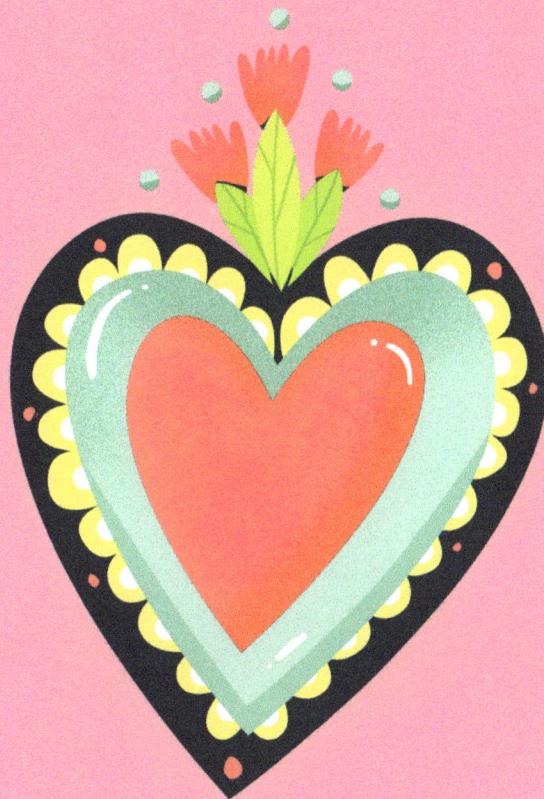

el corazón

the heart

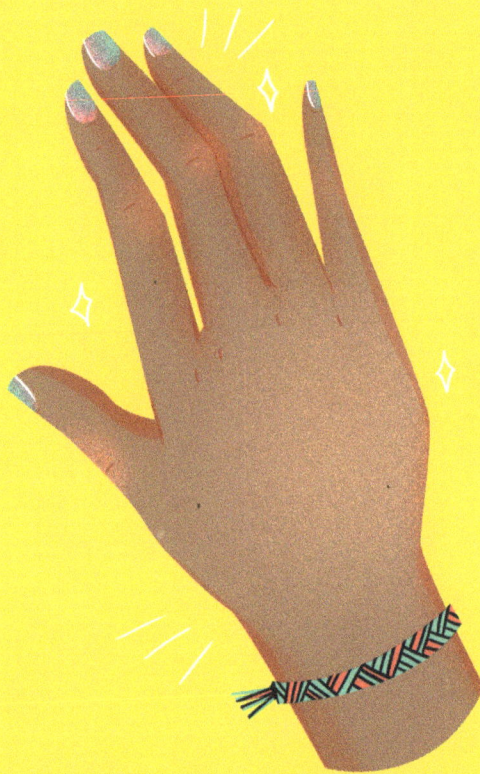

la mano
the hand

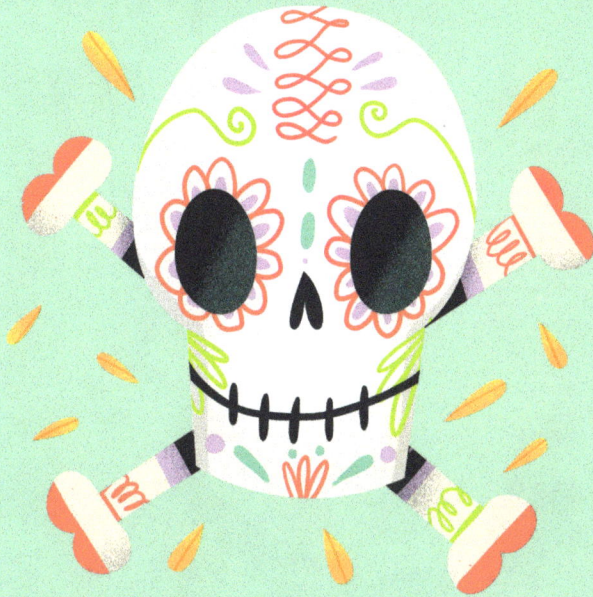

la calavera

the skull

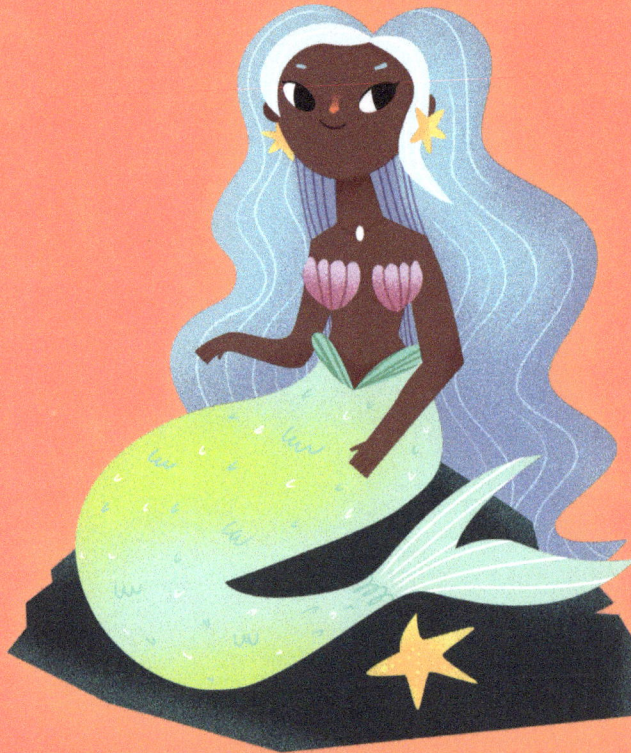

la sirena

the mermaid

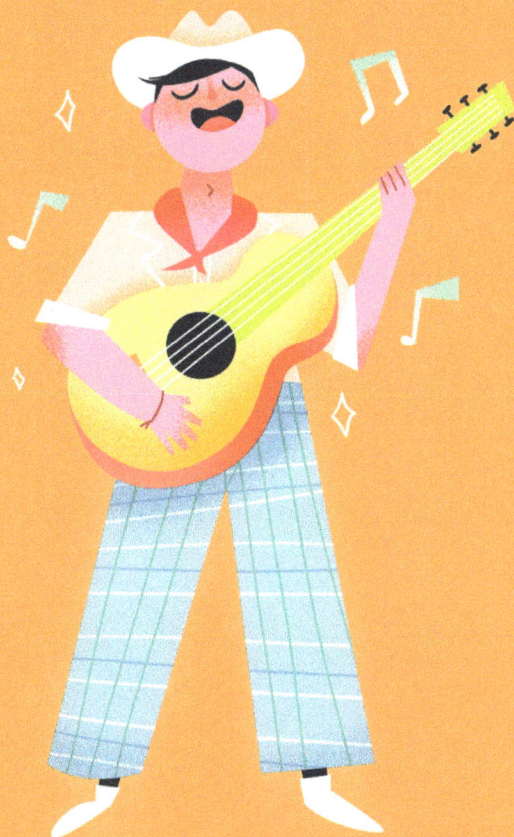

el músico

the musician

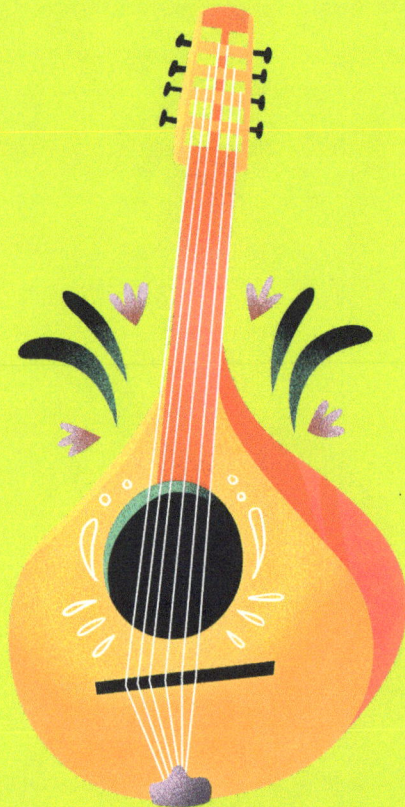

el bandolón

the mandolin

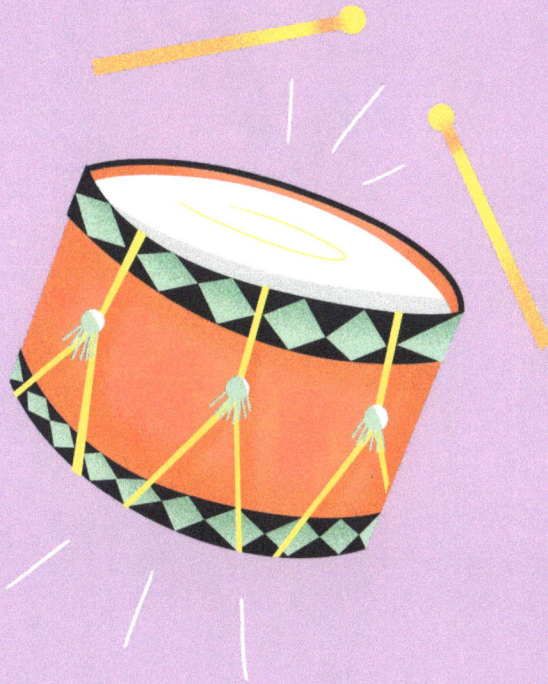

el tambor
the drum

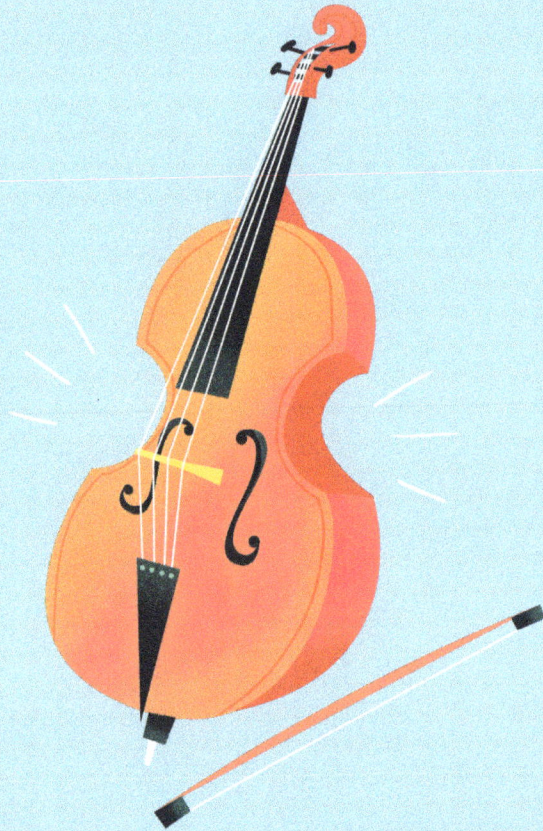

el violoncello

the cello

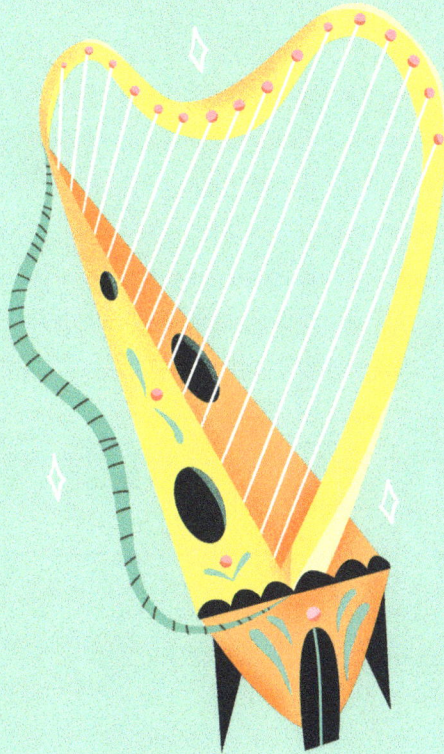

el arpa
the harp

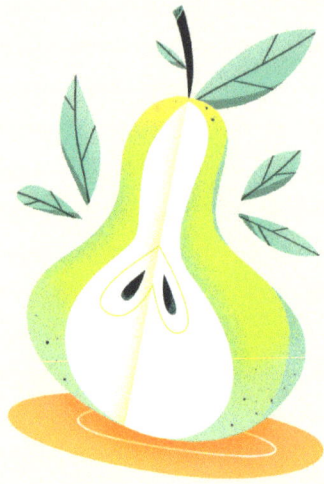

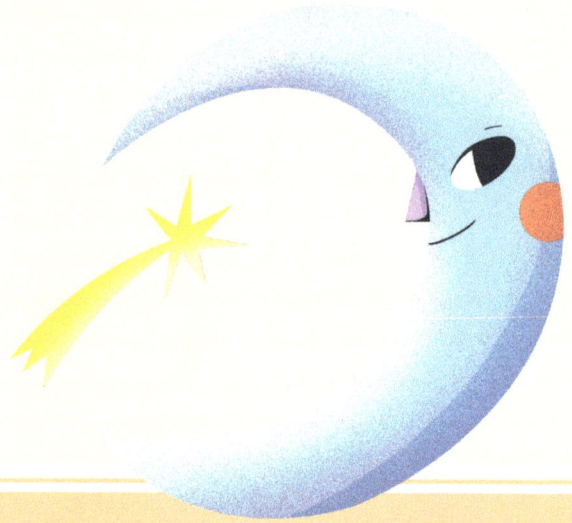

La naturaleza
The Natural World

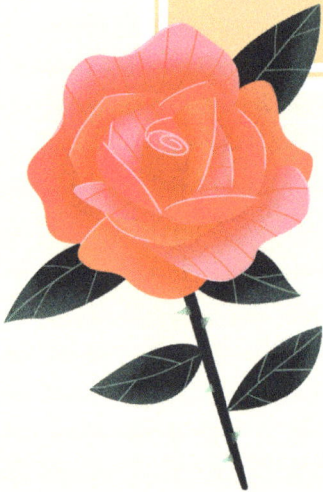

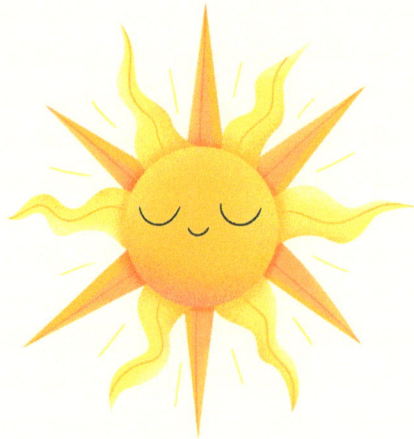

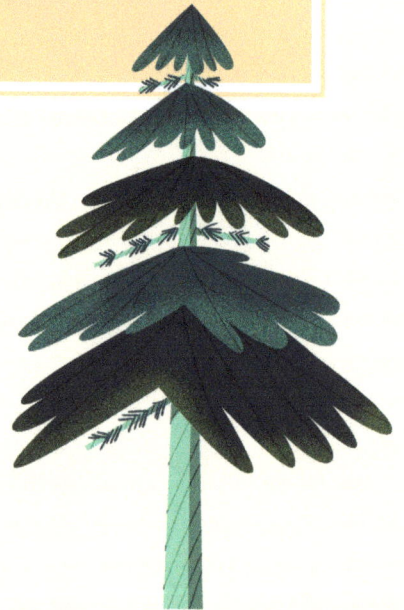

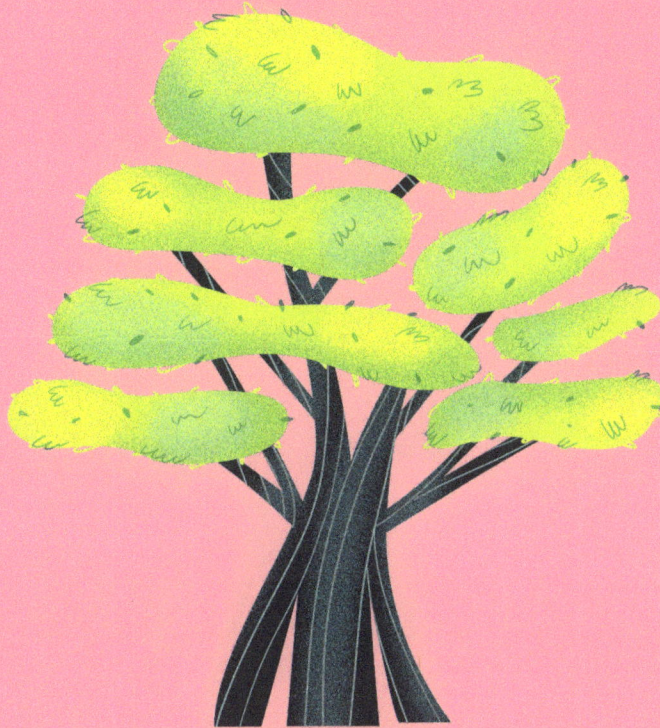

el árbol

the tree

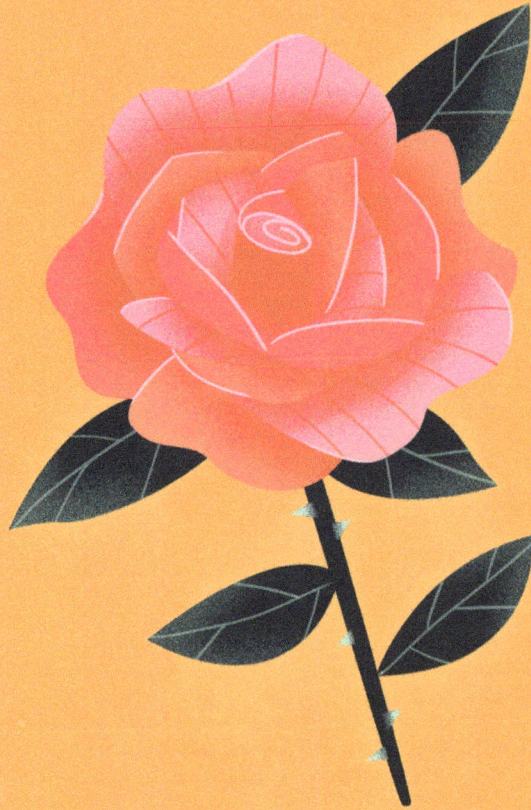

la rosa

the rose

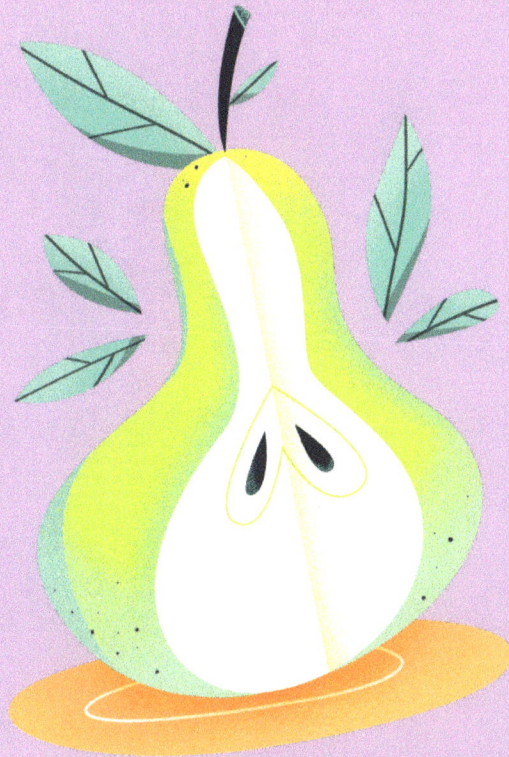

la pera

the pear

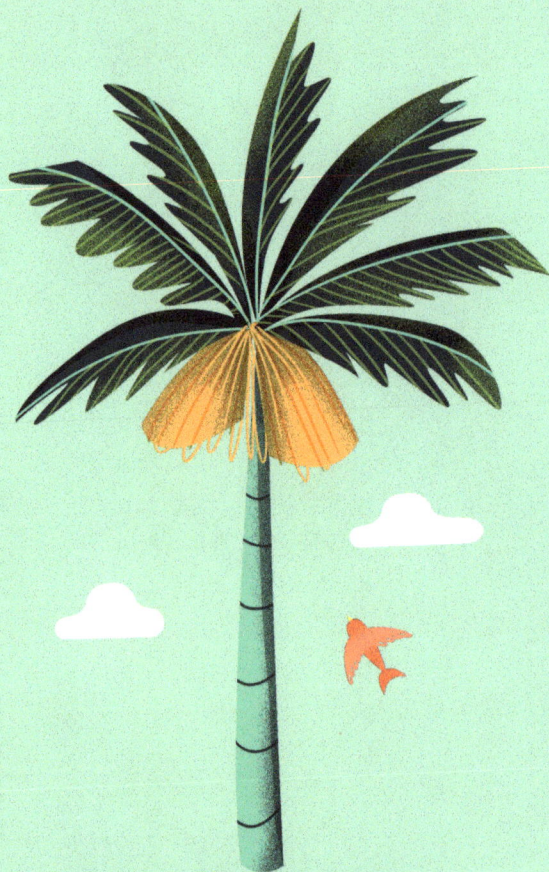

la palma

the palm tree

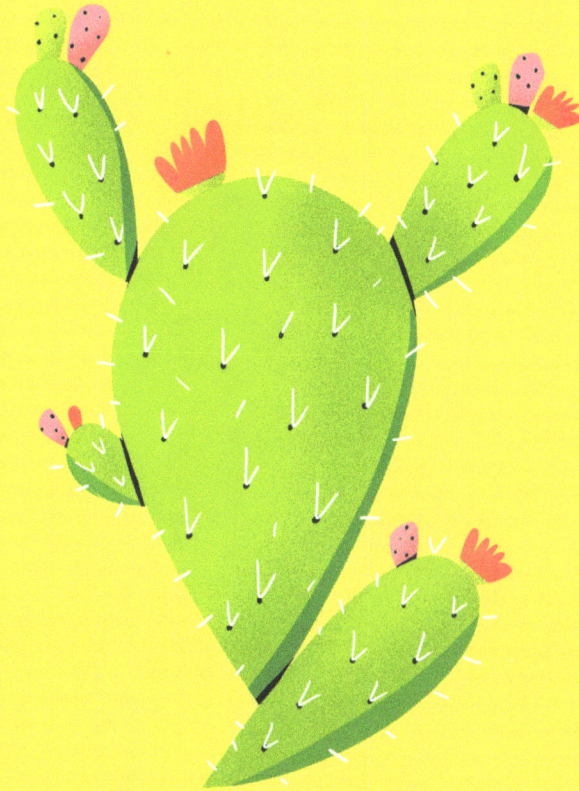

el nopal
the prickly pear cactus

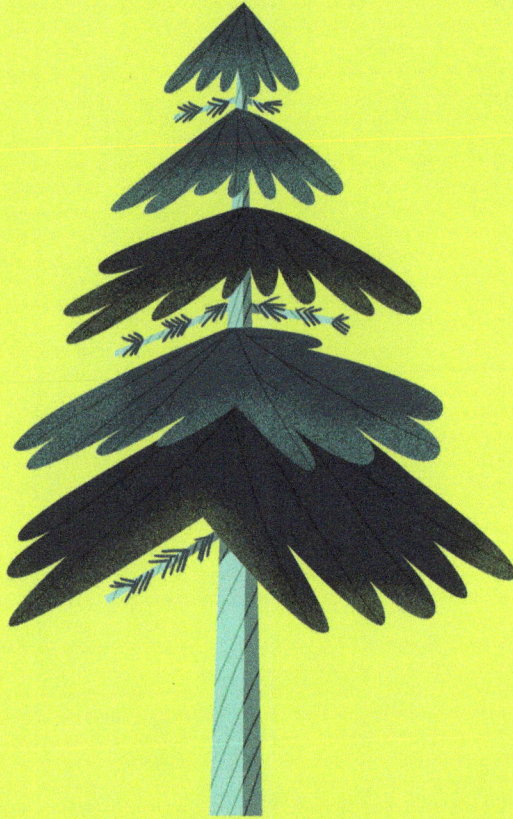

el pino
the pine tree

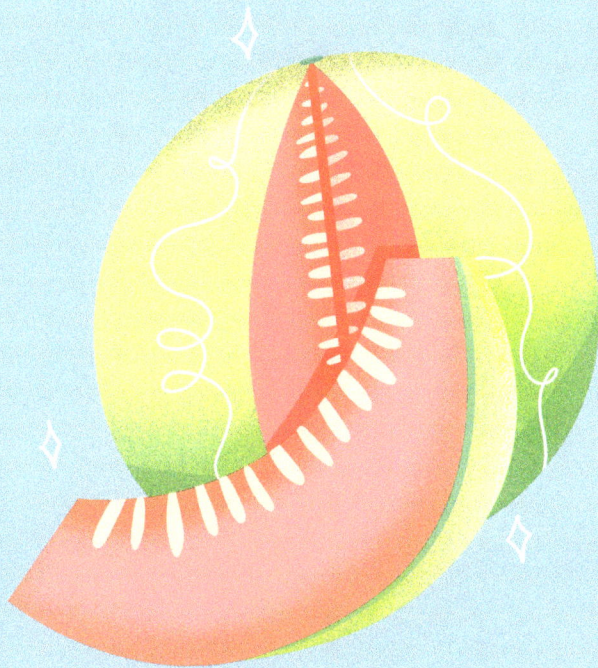

el melón

the cantaloupe

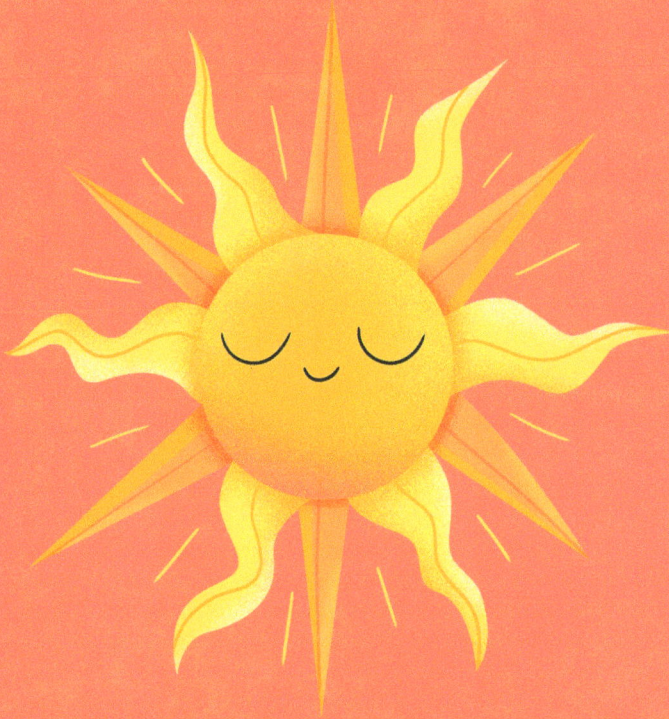

el sol

the sun

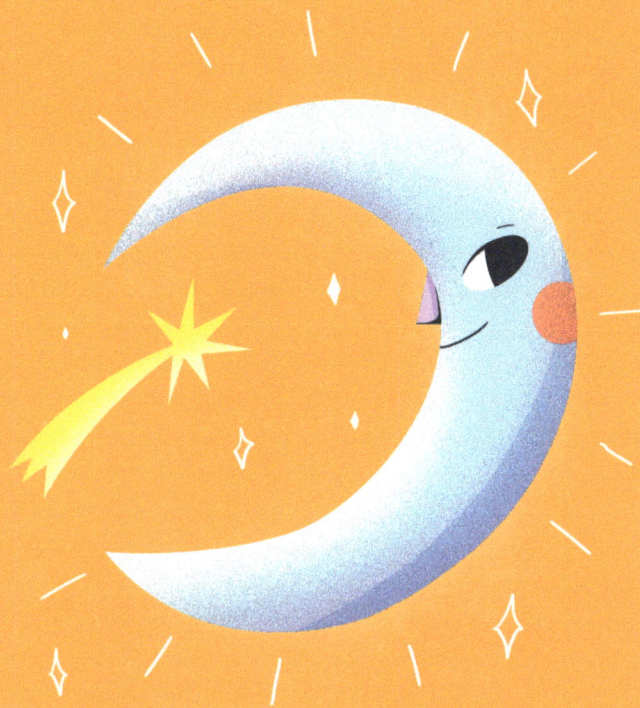

la luna

the moon

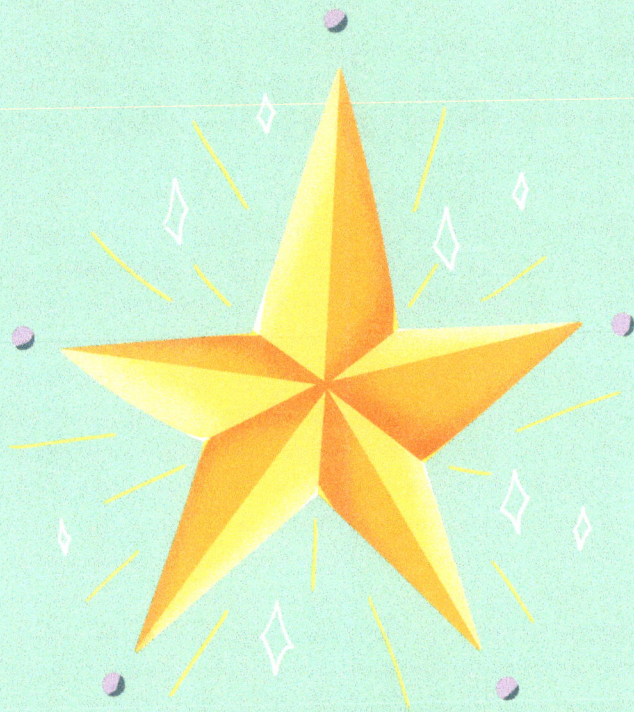

la estrella

the star

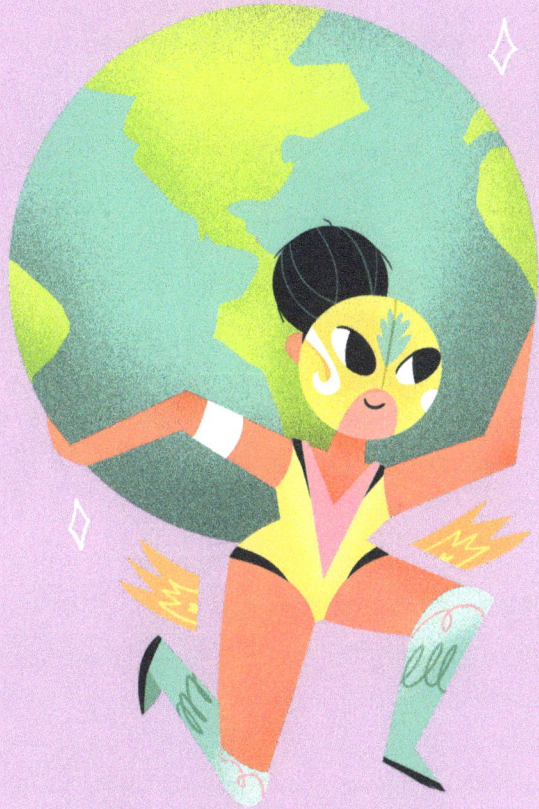

el mundo
the world

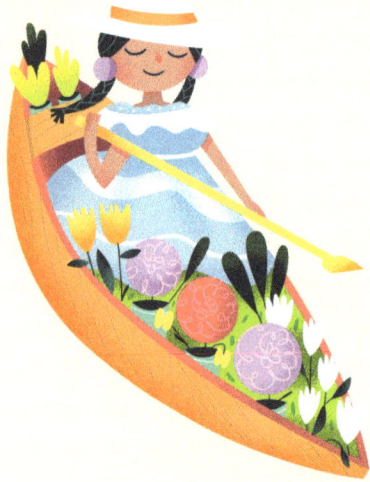

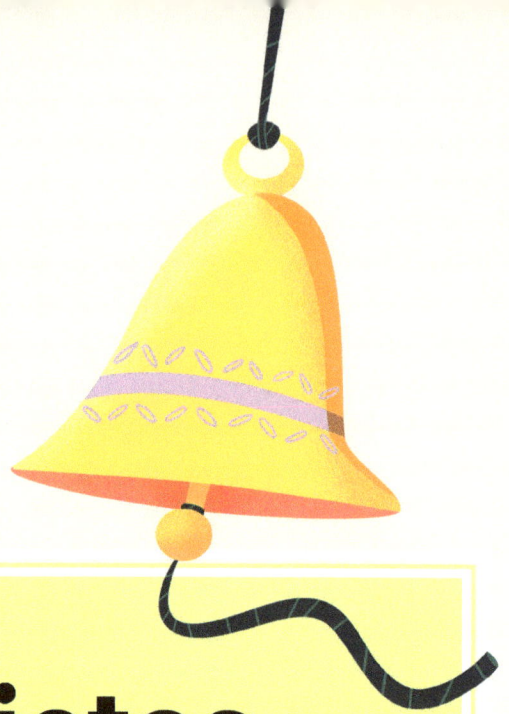

Los objetos
Objects

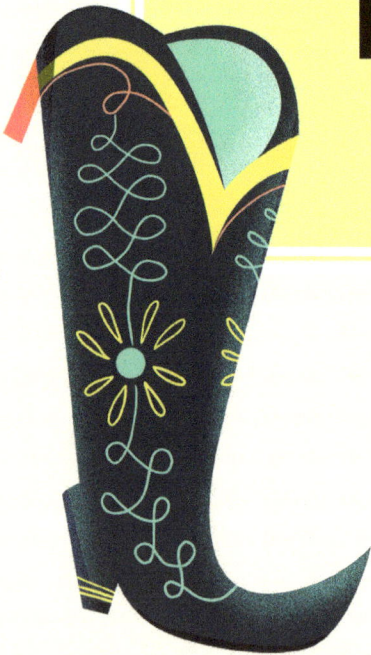

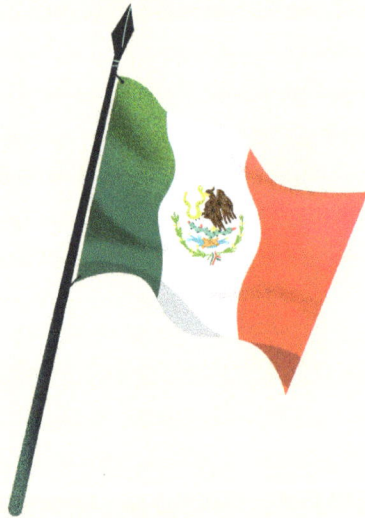

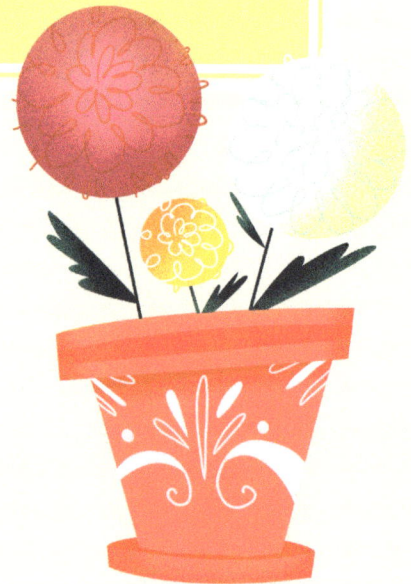

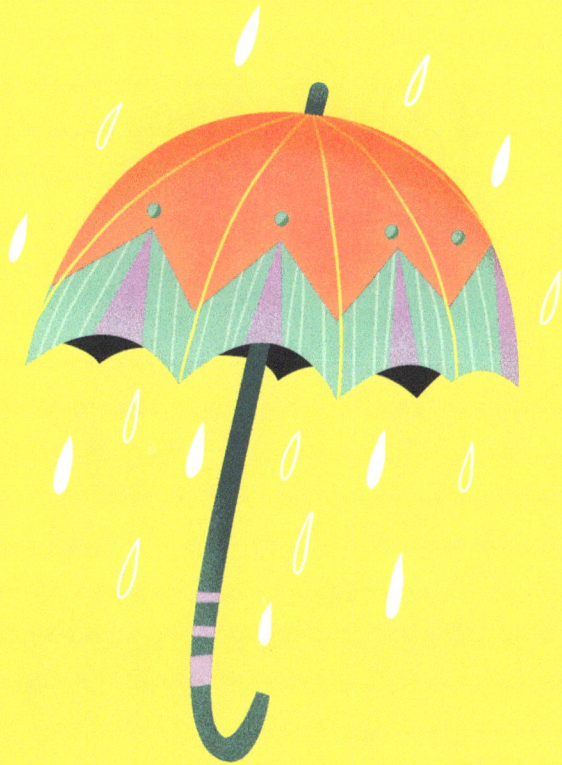

el paraguas
the umbrella

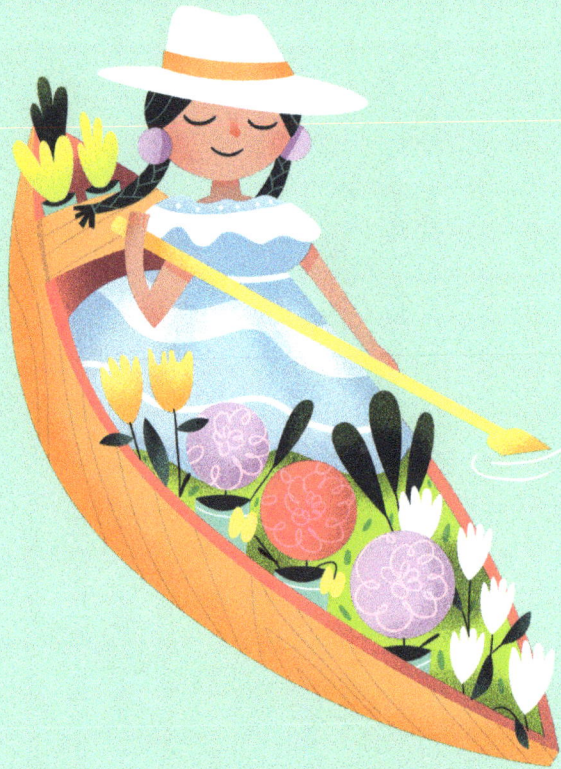

la chalupa
the canoe

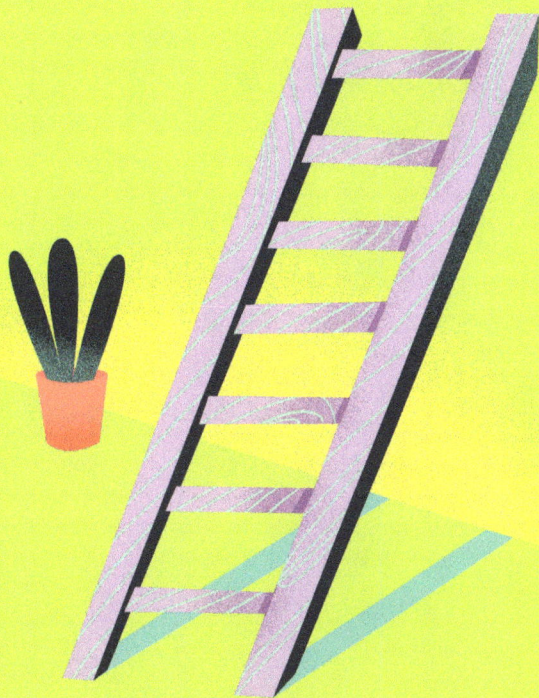

la escalera

the ladder

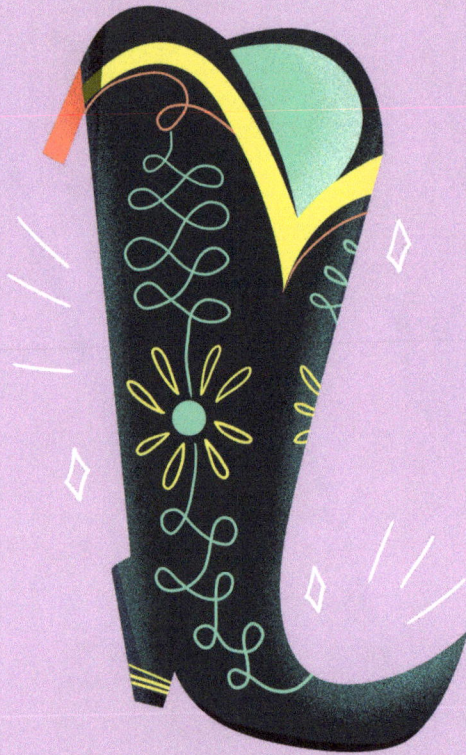

la bota
the boot

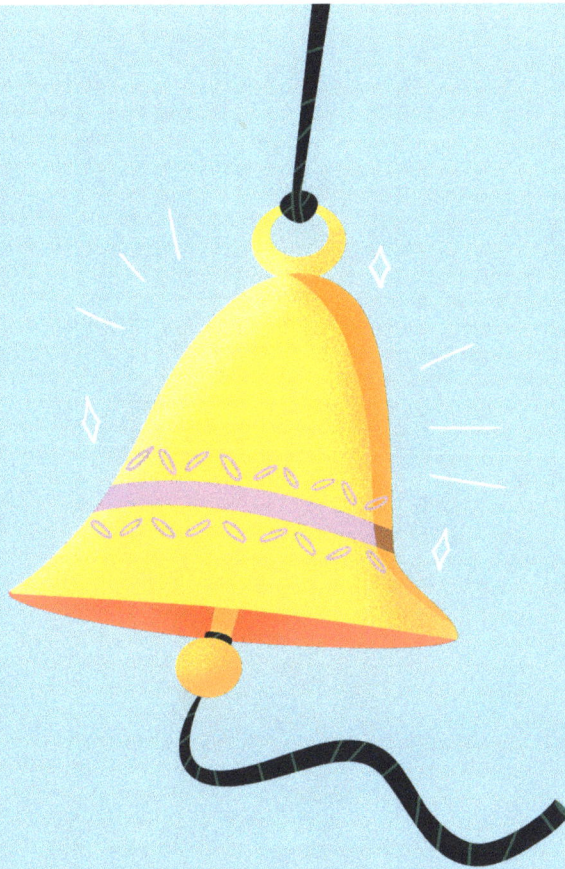

la campana

the bell

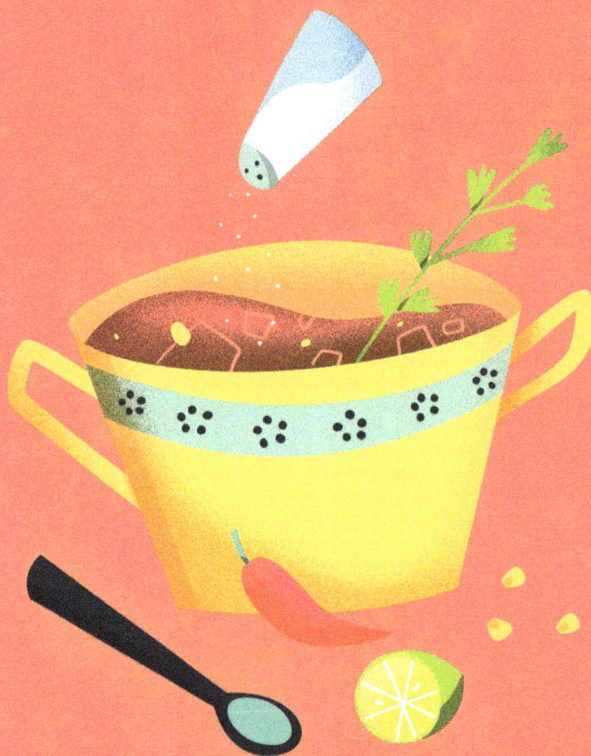

el cazo

the pot

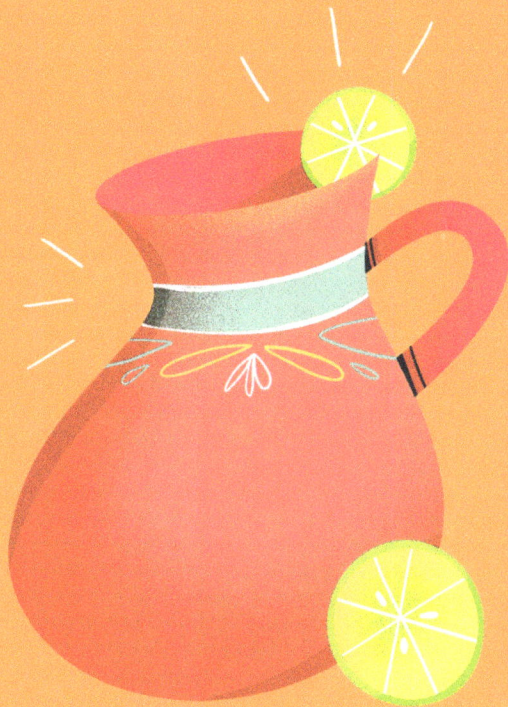

el cantarito

the pitcher

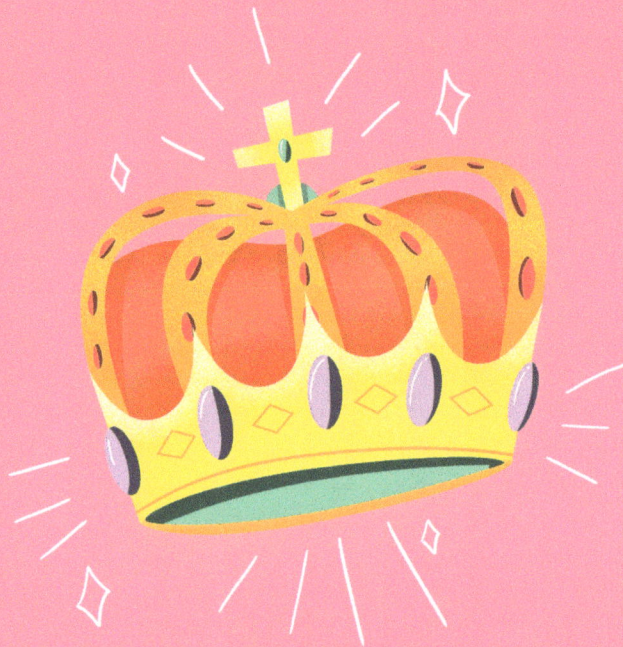

la corona
the crown

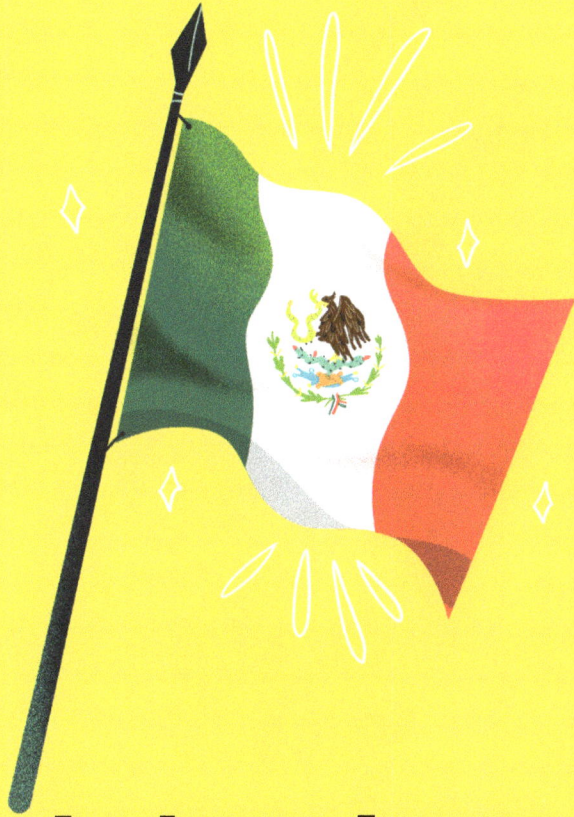

la bandera

the flag

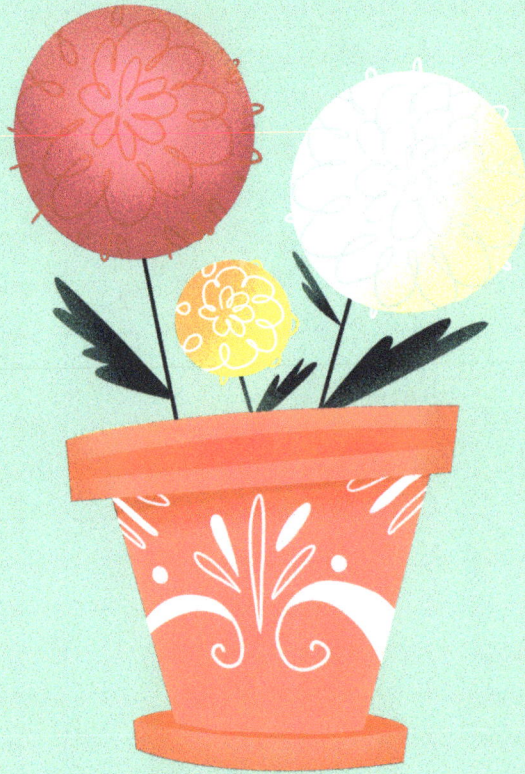

la maceta

the flowerpot

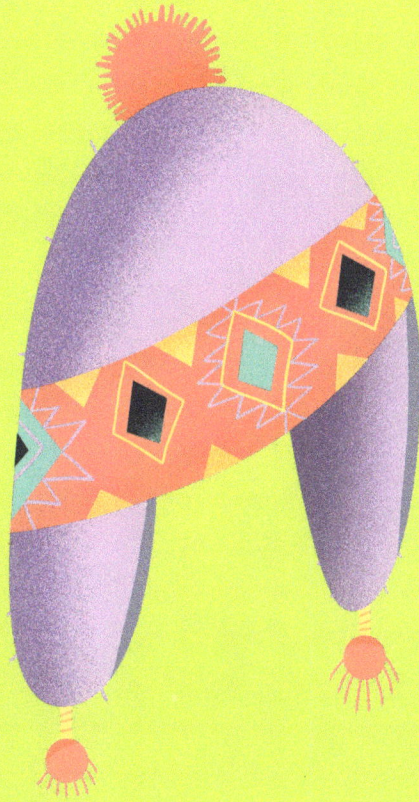

el gorrito

the hat

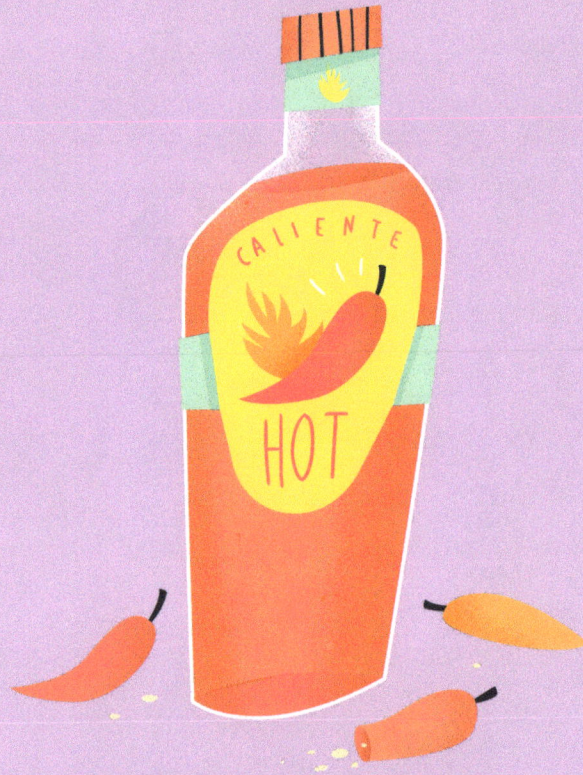

la botella

the bottle

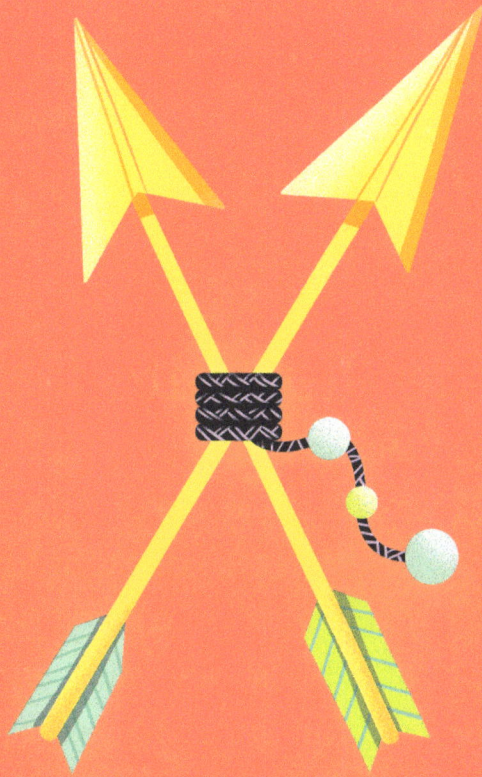

las jaras

the arrows

About the Author

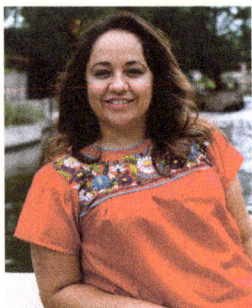

Angélica López is a teacher in Texas. She has spent the last eight years teaching English and Spanish in a dual language classroom for students in the lower grades. She is a wife and the mother of three very active boys. In her spare time, she loves to draw. This is her first book.

About the Illustrator

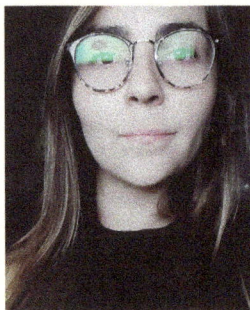

Milena Vargas (Muysuá) is a Colombian designer based in Mexico City since 2010. As an image lover she takes the time to reflect about how to reinvent word meanings through illustration. Her style is versatile, warm, and personal, colorful, and rich in details and textures that create emotion through each symbol and line she creates. She also works at Landor & Fitch México as a motion designer. She has worked for Discovery Networks, HBO Latin America, and Plaza Sésamo. You can see her work at instagram @muysua or on behance.net/muysua.

www.ingramcontent.com/pod-product-compliance
Lightning Source LLC
Chambersburg PA
CBHW051310020426
42331CB00019B/3496